No More Perfect Diets

My Experience with the Search for Perfect Heath

By Joey Lott

www.joeylotthealth.com

Publishing services provided by 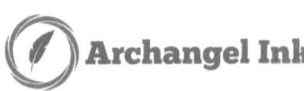 Archangel Ink

ISBN: 1518666116
ISBN-13: 978-1518666117

Table of Contents

The Descent into Perfection

I wanted perfect health. I wanted to avoid pain and sickness. Ultimately, I wanted to avoid death.

I was searching for the perfect diet for decades. I tried a lot of them. You probably have too.

Ultimately, none of the diets worked for me. In fact, the harder I tried and the longer I tried, the sicker I became. Eventually, I was desperately searching for the perfect diet to repair all the damage that my search for perfect health had inflicted.

Along the way, there were countless experts who assured me that their diet was the best. Whether it was raw vegan or low carb paleo or anything else, the experts sold their product well. I believed. I was a convert. I dived in with both feet.

I wanted to believe, because what they promised was nothing less than eternal happiness. Oh, sure, they didn't say that, precisely. They just talked about how the "perfect" diet would make me "vibrant" and "radiant." They just talked about how following all of their recommendations would make me "clean" and "detoxified."

But I could read between the lines. What they were really saying was that they had the solution to all of my problems. They held the secret to everlasting health. They knew how to stomp out sickness and death.

And, frankly, I was ripe for the deceit, because I was unhappy. Sure, I was on top of the world in some ways. I made good money. I practiced yoga every day. I had friends.

Yet I also had a dirty secret. I was terrified of feeling most feelings. I didn't want to feel the buzzy, high-strung feelings of anxiety. I didn't want to feel the shaky feelings of nervousness. I didn't want to feel the rising feelings of anger. Really, I only wanted a very narrow set of feelings. Just the small handful of feelings that I had deemed as "good."

I had been desperately trying to keep my experiences within this neat little grouping of allowable feelings through a variety of means. Food was my primary strategy.

I had been anorexic since a young age. I was certain that I needed to lose more weight and exercise more in order to shape my body in a way that I could accept. Over time, I lost sight of the original motivations for the restrictive eating, and it just became its own monster designed to keep feelings under control.

So even though I didn't always exhibit perfect anorexia symptoms, I was always restricting in some way. Eventually, this led to a decade's long succession of attempts to find the most perfect and pure diet imaginable.

I wanted the diets to work, but they never did. Oh, maybe here and there I'd experience some ups along the way, but then I'd crash. Over the years, my health declined.

The more my health declined, of course, the more this fueled my search for the perfect diet. So when some new diet would catch my fancy, I'd be a sucker for the promises of optimal nutrition, boundless energy, and so on.

Finally, however, after being incredibly sick for years, I had the good fortune to recognize that the search for the perfect diet was ruining my health. Upon discovering that, I embarked upon a process of undoing the restriction that I had placed upon my life. For me, this led to a remarkable rediscovery of health and well-being. My hope is that my story and the insights that I gained may prove helpful to you. I hope that something of my story will resonate with you and save you from some of the mistakes and the pain that I experienced.

Of course, I don't have all the answers to the dietary and nutritional puzzle, so never take my word for it. I simply want to share my experiences and the knowledge I have gained so that you can make better decisions. I don't have all the answers, and my hope is to demonstrate to you that they don't have all the answers either. There's nothing wrong with gathering advice from various sources. However, I sincerely hope that after reading this, you will have a more open mind and are more willing to listen to your own body's needs instead of the dietary advice of the self-proclaimed experts.

The Importance of Metabolism

For me, what finally turned things around was eating way more food than I thought I needed. This turned out to be very important for me, because I learned that undereating slows metabolism, and lowered metabolism has a lot of very unpleasant symptoms. Eating enough can reverse the problem.

I tell you this because I want to be clear with you from the outset that I necessarily am sharing my story with a bias; what helped me free myself from the vicious cycle of searching for the perfect diet was eating enough and removing the restrictions. And I have communicated with many other people who have experienced the same. Will this be the answer for you? I don't know for sure, but it seems like a very good possibility if you have been eating in a restricted way.

You name it, I've probably tried it. Vegan. Raw vegan. Paleo. Raw paleo. Sprouted grains. Grain free. Low fat. No fat. High fat. Sugar free. Salt free. Autoimmune protocols. Low carb. Zero Carb. And on and on.

All the experts assured me that they had the one true answer that would solve all my problems. If only I would eat the way they suggested (or insisted), then I would surely enjoy perfect health. They offered research and anecdotes and all kinds of evidence to support their claims.

Looking back on it now, much of the evidence was sketchy from the start. Yet some of it still remains convincing - theoretically, that is.

They would talk about protein, fat, carbohydrates, cholesterol, insulin response, fiber, sugar, leptins, lectins, enzymes, raw or denatured, and on and on.

Yet what almost no one ever spoke of is the potential importance of eating enough food to support a healthy metabolism. Almost no one ever spoke of how a slowed metabolism can lead to a whole host of symptoms, such as the following:

- insomnia or disturbed sleep (often waking in the early morning with symptoms of high cortisol and/or adrenaline)
- depression
- anxiety
- food sensitivities or intolerances
- leaky gut
- irritable bowel
- edema or fluid retention
- intolerance to cold (and sometimes heat)
- cold hands and feet
- low or non-existent sex drive
- memory and/or cognitive problems
- dry skin, possibly rashes
- muscle and joint pain
- falling hair
- weight gain or weight loss (weight gain is more typical, but weight loss can result, particularly in chronic hypometabolic cases when a person has difficulty consuming enough food)
- frequent urination - particularly at night

- fatigue

And I don't recall a single instance in which anyone mentioned that following their perfect diet was likely to slow metabolism.

Then I came upon the work of three people: Ray Peat, Matt Stone, and Dr. Broda Barnes. Each of these three emphasized the importance of metabolism above all else - more important than macronutrients or micronutrients or any particular ideology. They also offered novel insights about how one might go about making positive changes to metabolic health.

To be clear, I am not suggesting that any of these three have a monopoly on truth either. In fact, they each have their own peculiar ideas that can lead to more restriction if interpreted through the lens of an eating disorder. In fact, Ray Peat's work is notorious for fueling restrictive behaviors among those who want to believe, so I am not suggesting that anyone should look to any of these three to offer perfect guidance for the perfect diet. Rather, these three people's work opened my mind to the possibility that I had been wrong.

Furthermore, these three offered some useful insights into some diagnostics that one can use to measure metabolic health. They also gave some guidance as to how one might generally go about improving metabolic health. Without turning the information into a new ideology, I simply began to make observations of my own health and my own body, and I made adjustments to see what effect those adjustments had. Through some experimentation, I soon discovered greater health than I had experienced since my youth.

The simple diagnostics that I learned are basal temperature and resting pulse. If either is low, this is said to indicate low metabolism. I have found this to be true.

Basal temperature refers to temperature taken before arising from bed. If this temperature is under 98 degrees Fahrenheit or 36.5 degrees Celsius, then this is said to indicate low metabolism.

I never bothered to take basal temperature. Basal temperature is the lowest of the day, which is why it is best for measuring as a diagnostic. However, my morning temperature even after getting out of bed was consistently under 97 degrees Fahrenheit, so I already knew that my temperature was low.

Resting pulse is your heart rate when you have been resting. The ranges for healthy resting pulse vary depending on the "expert." However, combining the ranges, we get a range from 65-90 beats per minute, so the suggestion is that anything under 65 beats per minute is indicative of low metabolism.

Either a low temperature or a low pulse is suggestive of low metabolism. In my case, both were low. Yet if you have either a low temperature or a low pulse and you have any of the symptoms of low metabolism, then it seems likely that low metabolism may be in effect.

Once I had determined that low metabolism was likely a problem, I needed to know what to do about it. Again, I looked to the advice of the three who had offered help for diagnosing low metabolism, and I found that the fundamental advice is quite simple: eat enough.

How much is enough? What I discovered is that there is at least some good evidence that maybe "enough" meant a lot more than I had thought. Through some research, I discovered that some studies had been done to measure how much people actually eat instead of how much they report that they eat. The results showed that people actually eat considerably more than what they report. Since much of the standard recommendations are based on reported amounts, it seemed sensible to consider the possibility that I had been undereating.

What the studies show, more or less, is that healthy people eat approximately the following:

- males under the age of 25 eat 3500 calories a day
- males aged 25 and over eat 3000 calories a day
- females under the age of 25 eat 3000 calories a day
- females aged 25 and over eat 2500 calories a day
- pregnant and lactating women eat 3500 calories a day

So I decided to give this a fair trial. As I am male and over 25, I decided to commit to eating at least 3000 calories a day.

This turned out to be enlightening.

When I started counting calories, I found that I had been consistently undereating rather severely for years, even when I wasn't trying. I had restricted amounts of food consciously only for relatively short periods of time in my life - months at a time. Otherwise, I had never intentionally restricted the amounts I was eating, but simply due to the restrictive nature of the diets that I followed - meaning the limitations on the types of foods - I was generally undereating. And it was worst when I was trying to eat healthfully.

In fact, often times I had felt that I was gorging myself, and yet I was barely eating 1600 calories in a day!

So I realized that in order to do my experiment successfully, I was going to need to let go of some of my rules. I had to let go of my fear of dairy, my fear of sugar, and my fear of carbohydrates in general.

I realized that my health was a mess, and I had exhausted the restrictive dietary spectrum.

I was finally willing to do something different. I decided that just for the purposes of the experiment, I would let go of some of my rules and eat a minimum of 3000 calories daily.

I started eating large amounts of whole milk, honey, and maple syrup in addition to other foods. I ate white rice and potatoes with lots of butter. I made ice cream to eat. I focused on high-calorie, highly-palatable (i.e. low fiber) foods.

And I started to feel better.

There's a line from a Bob Marley song (borrowed from Psalms 118) that says, "the stone that the builders refused will become the head cornerstone." In a secular context, this can be seen to be a simple statement of wisdom regarding the human experience. We often reject that which is needed, and so eventually we come to discover that need and allow for that which we had rejected.

I had rejected carbohydrates and sugar. I had rejected low-fiber and refined foods. I had rejected adequate protein. I had rejected adequate calories. I had rejected food in general.

And when I invited enough food into my diet without all the restrictions of the past, my health improved. I started to sleep better. I started to have more stable moods. I started to have more energy. I started to gain strength without trying. My digestion (which had been a mess with all kinds of sensitivities and bloating) started to improve. Anxiety decreased. Hypersensitivity to all sorts of things started to decrease.

Is eating enough a panacea? No. But in my case, it sure came pretty close. I had so many health problems that seemed disparate. I couldn't make sense of them all, and the harder I tried to make sense of them, the worse they got…until I started to eat enough. Then I felt better. Much better.

I'm not alone in this, either. Since making this massive turnaround in my health, I have communicated with many others who have discovered similar improvements in health when ditching the unnecessary restrictions.

Does this mean that doing the same will solve your health problems? No, it is not guaranteed, but it does suggest a possibility.

And it is one that I personally can recommend exploring rather heartily.

The Importance of Letting Go

I very definitely had highly disordered eating habits going back to childhood. I know that I had gone through periods of extreme restriction and fasting to the point where I was dangerously emaciated, and I know that I had extreme anxiety about all things related to food. In fact, I even had paranoia - concerns about people tampering with my food to harm me. Because of this, I had no problem accepting that I had a problem. It was obvious.

You may know that you have an eating disorder, or you may not. You may be in denial. However, if the very idea of letting go of restriction frightens you or provokes anxiety, then this is a pretty good indication of disordered eating patterns. Of course, I cannot know if you have an eating disorder - only you can know that - but I will make some suggestions to you that may help you determine this for yourself.

Do you restrict food (types or quantities) in any way, even if you rationalize it as a pursuit of perfect health? Do you limit calories below the minimums that I listed earlier in an attempt to lose weight or feel better? Do you follow a restrictive diet, such as vegan, primal, paleo, Atkins, ketogenic, low carb, grain free, gluten free, dairy free, sugar free, low fat, or any other similarly-restrictive diet, without clear evidence of acute allergic reactions to the foods that you restrict? Do you think about food often? Do you read many books or blogs or articles about food? Do you have to prepare special meals for yourself? Do you feel that if you could only find the right diet, then everything would be okay?

If you answered yes to any of those questions, then please consider the very real possibility that your eating habits may be disordered, and this may be hurting you. It's not that there's anything morally wrong with disordered eating, so you don't have a moral obligation to change anything. Rather, it's just that your eating habits and, more importantly, your attitudes and beliefs about food and your body and health may be harming you and causing you to feel bad.

Because food is the focus of any eating disorder, it is easy to make the mistake of thinking that it is all about food. It is not. In my own experience and in my communications with others who have experienced disordered eating, food is only part of the problem. Anxiety and a desire to avoid certain thoughts and sensations fuels much of the problem that manifests as having to do with food.

To be clear, food is a big part of the problem. Eating too little is a problem if you want to have good health, and it is unreasonable to expect to feel well long-term without eating enough. However, it is only part of the problem.

The anxiety, fear, and other emotional components to disordered eating form the other part of the problem. In my experience, eating enough consistently tends to greatly diminish these parts of the problem. Eating too little lowers metabolism, which causes chronic stress in the nervous system, exacerbating anxiety, fear, obsession, compulsion, and the like. Yet here we have a bit of a catch-22, because the anxiety, fear, obsession, compulsion, and so on often make it seemingly impossible for a person to eat enough since they serve as triggers to restrict.

So if you experience any anxiety, fear, obsession, compulsion or other similar problems in regard to food, then perhaps my own story will be helpful to you.

I had long-standing problems with anxiety. Major anxiety. Anxiety so intense that I was eventually washing my hands compulsively, counting and doing other mental games to try and "cancel out" unwanted thoughts or sensations, and so forth. In fact, this anxiety drove me to move out of conventional housing and start living out of a van. I was a wreck.

Finally, what I realized was that I spent a lot of time thinking about problems and trying to resolve the problems, and yet the actual problem as I experienced it was a physical sensation. I am not suggesting that it was just one static sensation. Rather, I'm stating that I discovered that any time I found myself feeling anxious or stressed, I was in the habit of obsessing and fixating on thought as a way to try and solve the problem. Yet underneath all the thinking, I could find some physical sensation that I was actually feeling in the moment.

The focus on thinking and trying to solve the problem only kept the problem going. It was a vicious cycle. The more that I tried to solve the problem, the worse it got.

When I turned attention around, away from thought and toward the actual experience of the sensations, then I found that it was never what I had imagined it to be. It was a bit as though I had been running from the boogie man, but when I finally turned around to face the boogie man, he wasn't there.

I'm not suggesting that the sensation wasn't there, precisely. Rather, the sensation was never what I thought it to be. I would have a vague sense that the sensation was something to be avoided at all costs, like the boogie man. Yet upon turning and experiencing the sensation directly, I would invariably find that it was just a sensation.

That's the strange thing about sensations: they are just sensations. They have no inherent value or meaning. The value and meaning is all supplied by thought, which gives a story to the sensation. We give names and labels to sensations. We call them "good" or "bad." And yet, upon directly experiencing the sensation, it turns out to be just a sensation.

There is a biological basis for this phenomenon. The limbic system of the brain deals in emotion, and its primary function, it would seem, is to protect us from danger. In many cases, the limbic system performs superbly. The limbic system manages to move us out of danger's way without thought in many cases, and yet, we can inadvertently train our limbic system to perceive food or anything else as a life-threatening danger. When this happens, we can experience extreme panic, fear, and anxiety without any clear cause. So we have these strong sensations (emotions) that drive irrational behavior (such as self-starvation) and we have no idea why they occur. This is the limbic system doing exactly what it is designed to do. It's just that the limbic system has become hypersensitive, and if we want emotional health, then we need to reset it.

Eating enough tends to reset the limbic system in regard to food in two ways. For one thing, it physiologically resets the autonomic nervous system to parasympathetic dominance, which means a reduction in anxiety and fear. For another thing, by choosing to eat even when feeling anxiety or fear, this signals the limbic system that the anxiety or fear is not necessary in this type of situation, and so over time the limbic system adjusts accordingly.

Initially, the anxiety can prevent people from taking the necessary action (i.e. eating enough), so I suggest that if you find yourself in this situation, you may want to begin to practice some exercises to calm your limbic system and increase your emotional flexibility.

The simplest practice that I have found is to consistently turn your attention to direct experience of physical sensation whenever you find that you are thinking about a problem. There is no need to try and get rid of thoughts or change thoughts. Let the thoughts happen. Simply turn your attention to the direct experience of the physical sensation you feel in that moment. Don't give names or labels to the sensation. Just feel it and notice it without trying to get rid of it.

This simple practice has transformed my life in ways that are beyond the scope of this book to discuss. (I have written other books about this.) Suffice it to say that it has proven very effective in my life.

If you are interested in other practices that can help, then I encourage you to check out http://www.peacefulpossibility.com/, which is a site that I created with over three hours of free video training on techniques for letting go of stress and anxiety. It is an absolutely free resource that contains the best practices and information that I have discovered in many years of searching for answers.

Exploring the Diets

In the following sections, I will share with you my experiences with a variety of dietary ideologies that I followed over the years. I will share with you both my own experiences as well as some things I have learned about these diets that may shed some light on their limitations.

The bottom line is that none of these diets worked for me in the long term. And in my communications with others, I have yet to hear from anyone who tells me that these diets worked for them in the long term. True, some people experience some benefits from some diets in the short term or even sometimes for a few years. Yet after some time, these diets tend to be too restrictive. While many of them are appealing in theory (i.e. they sound nice), they don't usually deliver on the promises in the long term.

Will some of the diets work for some people in the long term? Maybe. That seems possible. And please understand that I am not trying to suggest that I am an expert on what is the best diet. I tend to believe that there is no such thing as a static optimal diet. I believe that learning to tune in to healthy body cues is the best approach. And while some of the research and ideas that come out of these various diets can be interesting or entertaining, I don't believe any of it typically works well as a substitute for listening to one's own body.

Low Fat

The low fat craze seems to have passed its peak, yet this way of thinking still persists. Low fat was my entry point into the world of special diets. It started when I was about 11 years old. I was a boy with breasts, and I had failed to get rid of my breasts through other means, so I finally concluded that they must have been due to too much fat.

This notion had been reinforced by my pediatrician, who told my mother that I was too fat. So I took hold of the latest fad - the low fat fad. I reasoned, as an 11-year-old would be likely to do, that dietary fat caused body fat and reducing dietary fat would reduce body fat. Of course, I was really only concerned with getting rid of my breasts, but I assumed that reducing dietary fat would work.

It didn't work, however, and so I became more fanatical about it. I reasoned that I needed to reduce fat more, so I cut out as much dietary fat as I could. I began to insist upon eating only foods that had nutritional labels on the packages that stated "no fat." My diet consisted largely of nonfat milk, nonfat cereal, nonfat canned vegetables, nonfat frozen vegetables, nonfat potatoes, nonfat rice, nonfat candy, and nonfat beans.

I became an adherent to the nonfat lifestyle. I cannot say that eating extremely low amounts of dietary fat ever produced any positive effects. However, I was committed to the *idea* of no fat, and so I stuck with this way of eating for the next six years.

I *did* lose weight initially. However, I suspect that was mostly due to intentional starvation rather than eating no fat, because during high school when I was relatively happy I ate unrestrictedly of nonfat foods, and I put back on a healthy amount of weight.

Although there are many pitfalls to the low fat/nonfat lifestyle, in retrospect I managed reasonably well. Fat is more than twice as calorie-dense as any other macronutrient, so theoretically one needs to eat far less fat than anything else in order to get enough calories. Or, put another way, one needs to eat more than twice as many grams of protein and carbohydrates as fat in order to get the same number of calories.

However, fat tends to be quite satiating (as is protein). Carbohydrates, particularly starch and sugar, are not so satiating, so in the absence of fat and while eating low protein (which I did), it is not difficult to eat enough calories from mostly carbohydrates. During high school, I would routinely eat massive amounts of sugar and starch. I would sometimes eat twenty bananas and five or six bowls of sugary cereal for breakfast. I would often eat just as much for lunch and dinner with snacks between, so I was probably averaging over 4000 calories a day.

The sheer number of calories I ate during that time would account for the amount of energy I had. I was able to play soccer and workout in the school gym. My sleep was wonderful. I would fall asleep and stay asleep for sometimes as long as ten hours at a time.

The problem with low fat or nonfat diets, apart from the restriction, is that fat would appear to be an important nutrient for most people. There are many vitamins that are fat soluble. That means that without adequate dietary fat, it is possible that over time one could end up with deficiencies of fat soluble vitamins.

In reality, no one knows for sure about this issue of fat soluble vitamin deficiency being caused by lack of dietary fat. It just seems like a likely theory.

I believe that I have personally experienced tremendous benefits from eating dietary fat, including improvements to my nervous system and tooth remineralization. (Many fat-soluble vitamins are thought to play an important role in shuttling vital minerals into bones and teeth.)

I now personally believe that there is good evidence suggesting that highly saturated fats, as are found in many animal fats, dairy fat, and some tropical oils, are very healthy. As they occur naturally in many of the foods that I enjoy eating - foods that taste good - then I naturally eat substantial amounts of saturated fats. I don't eat much polyunsaturated fat, because polyunsaturated fats occur in relatively low amounts in most of the foods that I desire to eat.

In other words, I let my taste be my guide. And it is working out well for me so far.

Veganism

My experiments with veganism overlapped with my nonfat experiments, so I have substantial experience both with low-fat/nonfat veganism as well as regular fat and high fat veganism.

I first converted to veganism around the time I was 13 years old. I honestly don't recall precisely what happened to lead to the conversion. I had rather logically eliminated meat from my diet simply because it was more or less impossible to find meat without any fat, so the only animal proteins that remained as options were nonfat milk and egg whites.

I was never a fan of egg whites, and without butter, they held little appeal. I *did* enjoy milk, even nonfat milk, however, so I don't recall why I gave it up. I suspect that it was due to some fear, but I don't know what it was precisely. I just know that by the time I entered high school, I had given up all animal proteins.

I recall an incident in which my father became very emotional about the whole thing. He did as was his custom, and he read a book on vegetarianism from the library as research. He sat me down and told me that he was afraid that I would die if I didn't eat enough protein, and he informed me that I had to at least combine grains and legumes to get complete proteins.

So I ate rice and beans as a staple during many of my vegan years.

In retrospect, veganism wasn't overtly terrible for my health in the short term. However, identifying with veganism was bad for my health since it provoked anxiety. I was always concerned about getting animal products in my food. In fact, I was fanatical about it. Like many vegans, I wanted strictly segregated food. I didn't want my "pure" vegan food to have ever touched anything that had touched animal products.

In the long term, however, I have concerns about veganism. In theory, it might work for some people., but I think that one cannot be too fanatical about being "healthy" when being vegan. Ironically, I believe that what really made veganism untenable for me was trying to eat "healthy" with lots of whole grains and beans and vegetables while limiting sugar and salt.

I also have genuine doubts about the quality of protein available in a vegan diet. Again, there are no rules that necessarily apply to everyone in every situation, but despite what I very much wanted to believe as a committed vegan, I now doubt that most plant proteins are truly adequate for humans. I don't know this for certain, of course, but I know for me personally, I feel *way* better when eating animal protein. I believe that particularly collagen/gelatin, which is an animal protein, has been extremely helpful for me, and others report similarly.

Another important component of the vegan lifestyle is that it is meant to be concerned with animal welfare. I certainly know that during many of my years as a vegan this was a big part of my rationale for my choice.

What I have discovered for myself, however, is that refusing to eat animals is not actually the same as preventing animal cruelty. In fact, for me, using veganism as a shield of righteousness blinded me to reality as it is. The reality, as I now see it, is that death happens, and that death often happens in ways that seem horrific. Refusing to eat meat does not stop that.

I don't personally like factory farms, so I prefer to get animal products either from animals that I have raised or from farms that give the animals access to the outdoors and a natural diet whenever possible. This is a personal choice, of course, and I don't extend my preferences as a sort of imposition onto others. My point here is simply that if ethical choices are important to you, then it is possible to make ethical choices while eating animal products.

I do understand that many committed vegans feel there is no way they can ever eat meat or other animal products. That is fine. I have no need to convince anyone of anything.

I am merely offering insights from my own experience. If it resonates with you, great. If not, then that is fine too.

However, if you are vegan and your health and happiness are suffering, you may find that opening your mind to the possibility that you have been seeing the situation narrowly may be helpful to you. It was helpful for me when I realized that even growing carrots kills and displaces animals. It is noble to want to minimize the suffering of others, but to me it seems wise to see the bigger picture and recognize that death is a part of life. In doing so, my own experience is that it is possible to live in a way that truly respects life in a much larger way.

Raw Veganism

When I was 17 years old, I first encountered the idea of raw veganism. I was unhappy in life. I had found college to be a huge disappointment, and so I was looking for some way to feel better about life. I learned of raw veganism through some books by authors such as Ann Wigmore, Arnold Ehret, and Viktoras Kulvinskas.

The idea appealed to me in many ways. For one, it appealed to my desire for "purity" and "perfection." For another thing, it appealed to my search for specialness. It also appealed to my intellectual curiosity. When I thought about it, I concluded that a raw vegan diet made the most sense as the species-appropriate diet for humans. After all, I concluded, we surely must have evolved from earlier hominids who had not mastered fire or tools to be able to consistently hunt.

In the context from which I understood the situation, raw veganism seemed like the answer. The authors promised that raw veganism was the cure for everything from cancer to depression to spiritual confusion. It sounded like a panacea!

I really wanted raw veganism to work, but it didn't. Not even remotely. Granted, I took it to the extreme, but even upon subsequent experiments with raw veganism during which I was not so extreme, it never worked.

I tried raw veganism on multiple occasions over the years. I tried it in different forms. I tried sprouted grains, nuts, seeds, and legumes, and I tried without. I tried dehydrating food, and I tried without. I tried fermenting and without. I tried smoothies and without. I tried fruitarianism. I tried massive amounts of coconut. I tried lots of different variations.

None of it worked for me. I just ended up fatigued and exhausted. I lost weight. I felt spaced out. I felt anxious. I had insomnia. I got constipated.

And still I kept trying because all the experts said that my symptoms were just "detox symptoms."

Finally, however, I came to find that - at least for me - those weren't detox symptoms. They were symptoms of *too little food*.

I know that there are now those who advocate for eating massive amounts of calories on a raw vegan diet. Mostly, they advocate for a low fat raw vegan diet with carbohydrates from fruit as the primary energy source. This is called the 80/10/10 diet, which is popularized by the 30bananasaday.com website.

Although theoretically eating 4000 calories a day from fruit should provide enough energy, it doesn't seem to work very well. At several points in my life I attempted to eat in that fashion for some time, and it didn't work for me. I suspect that this way of eating does not provide enough quality protein or salt while simultaneously overloading the body with water.

Perhaps there are raw vegans who thrive long-term on such a diet. However, I honestly suspect they are few and far between.

Whole Food

Until my first stint with raw veganism (which ended horrifically with severe emaciation), I had eaten plenty of sugar and refined grain. However, after learning about all the supposed evils of sugar and refined grain, I decided to eat a whole foods diet.

So even though I gave up on raw veganism (until I returned to it the next time), I became committed to eliminating refined sugar and refined grain from my diet. This is when veganism began to cease working for me.

When I switched to a whole foods diet, I gave up on white rice, bread, or anything with added sugar. And although I didn't know it then, this forced me to eat less.

The reality is that whole grains add bulk while reducing usable energy by weight and volume. In other words, a cup of white rice is a more efficient energy source than a cup of brown rice.

Likewise, reducing sugar also reduced my energy intake.

So little by little, my energy declined.

I started practicing yoga (fanatically) in 2001. My energy slowly kept depleting over time until by 2006 I gave up on yoga almost entirely because I could barely get through a class any longer. I now attribute this depletion in energy to chronic calorie deficits coupled with increasing anxiety.

Whole foods are a nice idea. This diet appeals to the intellect. It certainly seems sensible that food would be best in its whole form, and when the advocates of whole foods tells us that refined foods are devoid of nutrients, this can be convincing. After all, we're told that the introduction of refined grains into diets lead to various diseases, such as beriberi, that are the result of nutrient deficiencies.

The problem is that cutting out all refined carbohydrates tends to lead to calorie deficits. So the ideology is nice, but it doesn't seem to lead to a sustainable practice.

Personally, when I began eating refined carbohydrates again in moderation (when I desire them) as well as sugar (including cane sugar!), my health started to improve. Of course, I cannot state that anyone else will see the same results. However, anecdotally, others have reported similar results, so I'm not alone in this.

There is so much propaganda in the air these days about how refined carbohydrates and sugar are the cause of so many problems. We are told that they are the cause of insulin resistant diabetes and other health problems, so I understand that letting go of the belief that refined carbohydrates and sugar are evil can be scary. All I can say is that the evidence is not all in favor of the presently prevailing theory that villainizes carbohydrates and sugar. Furthermore, my own experience runs counter to the propaganda.

I am not, of course, suggesting that you should eat tons of GMO bleached sugar as a new health food if it goes against your actual desires. In fact, hopefully you understand that I'm not suggesting that you *should* do anything. I'm merely offering you insights from my own experience, and in my experience, eating natural sugar (I have gone through phases of eating fairly massive amounts of honey, maple syrup, and cane sugar) has proven to be very helpful in restoring and maintaining health. The key, in my experience, is to eat what is desired. (Though initially, hunger cues and appetite may be sufficiently suppressed or imbalanced that monitoring for minimum intake is helpful.)

Paleo

I reached a breaking point in 2009. I had grown extremely unstable. I left my business. I moved into a van. And then I spent the winter at an outdoor school in northern Wisconsin.

The outdoor school provided all the food. What was available was meat, animal fat, non-starchy vegetables, and some limited starchy vegetables, so I broke my long-term vegan diet, and I began a mostly paleo diet.

"Paleo diet" refers to a popular diet that eschews any types of food that our paleolithic ancestors would not have likely eaten. While paleolithic people (meaning prior to agriculture) clearly wouldn't have eaten cultivated cabbage, the theory goes that they would have eaten similar sorts of plants. So cabbage is okay. Similarly, since paleolithic people would have eaten some starchy tubers, then sweet potatoes are generally accepted within paleo groups.

We are led to believe that paleolithic people would most certainly not have had access to significant dairy or grain. As such, these foods are strictly forbidden by most paleo diet enthusiasts. Of course, there are varying opinions within paleo groups, and certainly some will eat moderate amounts of grains or dairy, but generally, these foods are minimized.

The paleo diet theory is certainly interesting and curious. It is a compelling argument that humans survived for hundreds of thousands of years prior to agriculture, presumably eating no grain, no dairy (apart from mother's milk during infancy,) and no refined sugars. As such, it is reasonable to argue that this may well be the natural human diet.

However, in practice, it didn't work for me. In retrospect, the primary reason it didn't work was that it was darn near impossible to eat enough calories.

I ate lots of meat, broth, organs, and animal fat. I ate lots of vegetables. But it didn't add up to enough.

I see now how I could likely have modified the diet to make it work. Eating way more fruit and starchy vegetables could probably have helped, so I am not meaning to suggest that a paleo diet couldn't work.

However, I now question whether such a diet has any intrinsic value. Many of the arguments for a paleo diet suggest that grains and dairy are inherently problematic, but as with so many health topics, the evidence is mixed. There doesn't seem to be any overwhelming evidence that grain and dairy are problematic, and the reality is that grain and dairy are both easy and convenient sources of needed energy in modern life. Cutting them out removes many options for getting necessary calories.

During my paleo days, I was perhaps at my sickest. I was light-headed. I was severely emaciated. I was fatigued and exhausted beyond belief. I was horribly nauseous. I would wake up in the middle of the night with violent nausea followed by diarrhea.

And I kept believing that I just needed to find a better, more perfect diet to fix everything.

Low Carb

Atkins planted the notion of low carbohydrate in my head. I had never read Atkins, but I had plenty of acquaintances over the years who preached its tenets to me. So I got the idea stuck in my head. After paleo wasn't working out, I decided to investigate the idea of low carbohydrate paleo.

Turns out there's plenty of support for the idea. I found that Mark Sisson, author of *Primal Blueprint*, strongly suggested that a low carbohydrate diet could solve many health problems. Then I came across a website, healingnaturallybybee.com, that also suggested that low carb was the way to go, with lots of supporting evidence.

So I took the plunge. I went low carb. Eventually, I was eating only grass-fed meat and organs and fat, gelatin, egg yolks, apple cider vinegar, lemons, limes, cucumber, lettuce, parsley, and cilantro. I was terrified of anything else.

No matter how much I would eat, I could never eat enough to support a healthy metabolism. There just wasn't any way to eat enough of those things.

On the upside, I ceased to have the violent nausea after going low carb. However, nothing else improved.

Finally, I had reached a dead end. I just exhausted my ability to believe in the perfect diet any longer.

It was at that point that I encountered the work of the three people I mentioned earlier in the book - Ray Peat, Matt Stone, and Dr. Broda Barnes. I decided to experiment with eating with fewer restrictions and eating a minimum of 3000 calories a day. Only then did my health improve, including the horrible anxiety, insomnia, fatigue, food sensitivities, bloating, constipation, cold hands and feet, irritability, and so on.

What Does "No Restriction" Mean?

There is so much propaganda when it comes to diet that letting go of restriction can take some time. It tends to happen in layers.

I don't believe there is some ideal, "perfect" state of no restriction that one should strive for. Rather, I believe that the best guide is a) what is your state of physical health? and b) what is your state of emotional flexibility? If both are good, then there's no problem. If either is a problem, then it is worth exploring if there are any ways in which you find that you restrict your food or your experience based on belief or ideology (or fear), rather than on necessity.

With that said, my life improved when I let go of some key restrictions. I personally found that eating protein, fat, and carbohydrates unrestrictedly was essential. That meant quality animal protein, saturated fat, and both starches and sugars. Plus, salt turned out to be very important for me as well. I had simply been in the habit of using little salt. When I increased my salt intake significantly, my health improved tremendously.

I am not suggesting that these specific changes are likely to yield similar results in your life. I am merely suggesting that they are worth exploring.

The Traps of The Perfect Diet Promise

The advocates of the perfect diets make them sound so wonderful. They paint a picture of a utopia in which everyone who follows their rules will get to live in perfect health and happiness everlasting.

And they tend to back up their claims (not always, but often) with lots of scientific studies and peer-reviewed articles and the like, all of which lends a lot of credibility to their arguments.

The problem is that experientially, these diets simply don't work for a lot of people. Maybe they work for some, but not for all, and probably not even for most. Furthermore, even just logically, there is a problem that presents itself upon looking at the bigger picture: How is it that all of these conflicting diets could truly be the one true diet that will solve all of your problems? After all, raw veganism and paleo are rather fundamentally in opposition to one another, yet advocates of both claim that they have the one true diet. Vegan advocates claim that eschewing meat and animal products will give you everlasting health, while paleo advocates claim that animal products are essential for health! How can both be right?

In my own experience, the search for the perfect diet was an addiction. Others have confessed the same to me as well, so there are at least some of us who were searching for the perfect diet for reasons that blinded us to the bigger reality.

Of course, over time we had genuine health problems. No doubt about that. I was incredibly sick, and those health problems can fuel the search for the perfect diet. But the fact remains that, in my own experience, the stage was set such that no matter what other "genuine" factors may have contributed to the search, I was blinded to the bigger picture. I believed that I needed a restrictive, special diet. As such, that is what I kept finding.

For me, the answer came not from restricting, but by giving up the restrictions. The answer came from finally learning to let my body take care of itself. I didn't need to be the great dictator that kept tight control over my body. Instead, I discovered that there is an inherent intelligence in my body that can take care of itself when I get out of the way.

It was a process. It required resetting some systems. It required rediscovering intuitive cues. Yet over time, the outcomes have been entirely positive.

Will the same work for you? I don't know. I don't wish to speculate. There is certainly evidence suggesting that it is a possibility. Because of that, I would suggest that it is worth exploring, and only you can do that.

It seems that that is the way out of the trap of searching for the perfect diet: exploring for yourself. Discover for yourself. Instead of believing others, find out for yourself.

Everybody Is Going to Die

It may be possible to keep your physical form forever, but I doubt it. In fact, if you look closely, you'll notice that your physical form is never the same. My body today is not the same body as when I was two years old. In fact, it isn't even the same body as ten seconds ago.

Bodies are always changing, and from the best that I can tell, they die eventually. This is to say that some threshold is crossed in which the body no longer holds together under the organizing principle of individuality. Instead, the body is reintegrated into the greater whole.

When I was restricting, I was trying to hold on to some sense of being someone that I could defend and protect. I wanted to be me -

the me that I wanted to be. I wanted to be the safe, calm, okay me.

But finally, for me, there came the realization that this body will pass away. No matter what I attempt to do, this body will pass away. No matter how perfectly I eat or behave, this body will pass away. All bodies die, as best I can tell.

When I finally really let that in without resisting in any way, I ceased to be afraid. Discovering the reality of death ended my fear of death, and this allowed me to truly live. Strange, I know.

The reason that I share this is that in my conversations with others, I often hear a similar confession - fear of death driving the bus, so to speak. Others also report that upon finally fully allowing the reality of death without resistance, there is a peace and freedom that reveals itself.

In my experience, as long as I wanted to avoid death (and pain, which I'll mention in a moment), I was susceptible to the perfect diet claims. Yet upon truly accepting the reality of death, those claims ceased to have any appeal to me.

We all naturally want to avoid pain and sickness. That is fine, but in my experience, there is no sure way to avoid these things. I am sure we all know or know of people who have lived perfect and pure lifestyles and yet died of cancer at a young age. And we all know or know of people who have eaten fast food and smoked cigarettes while living reasonably healthy lives until they died peacefully at age 90.

My experience is that when I finally accepted the reality of death, I discovered that no one has a monopoly on truth. In fact, perhaps the only truth of which we can be certain in this sense is that no one absolutely knows anything. There is evidence to support particular beliefs, of course. And relatively-speaking, some of that may seem to hold true. Smoking cigarettes does tend to correlate to lung cancer, for example. And yet, correlation does not suggest causation. It could be purely coincidence. Or there could be other causes that are hidden to us.

Not, of course, that I am suggesting that anyone should smoke cigarettes and eat fast food if they don't want to. I'm just saying that despite what we think we know, we don't actually know.

And so nothing that I state in this book should be taken as a new belief. I don't know anything either. It's just that now I know that I don't know, and this seems to be much healthier.

In recognizing that I don't know, I no longer try to control my body. I trust in the inherent intelligence of my body to take care of itself. And while I am certainly willing to experiment and try out various ideas and theories if they seem appealing or interesting and appropriate, I do so lightly and easily. I have no major investment in those things. If something doesn't make my body feel good, then it is a clear indicator that it's not right at the moment.

Things are greatly simplified. Eat when hungry. Rest enough.

There was an intermediate period in which I had to adapt to trusting my body. It was a process. For me, I committed to eating at least 3000 calories a day for a few months, and I committed to challenging myself to eat foods that I felt anxious about yet knew were not real threats.

Eventually, I found that I rediscovered hunger cues and other bodily signals that I had completely suppressed or misunderstood previously. Since then, I simply trust my body. If I am hungry, I eat. If I desire something particular, then I eat that. If not, then I just eat something. It's no longer a big deal.

Strangely, now that eating isn't such a big deal, it is far more enjoyable. I no longer think about food. I just eat food, which is a wonderful experience. I used to think about food instead of eating. Even when I was eating, I was layering on thought as a mediator. Now I directly experience the actual eating, and this is sometimes quite pleasurable. Still, it's not a big deal.

What Now

My hope with this book is that I can offer you something that will open your mind to the possibility of something beyond your current belief system. If your health is less than optimal and you've been searching for the perfect diet, then I invite you to explore this more deeply. Instead of trying to figure it all out, see if it may be possible that it's much simpler than you have thought it to be. What if, after all, your body has the intelligence within it to know what it most needs? And what if your body can take care of itself? What if you don't need to agonize over what to eat?

Get My Future Books FREE

If you enjoyed this book (Hey, if you made it this far it couldn't have been that bad), you'll probably enjoy many of my other books about health and wellness. And you can get all my new releases in health and wellness for free by signing up for my mailing list at www.joeylotthealth.com. It's simple, it's free, and it's totally honest and legitimate. Nothing scammy or spammy or anything else like that (i.e. I won't be trying to sell you The 7 Dirty Underground Top Secret Weird Tricks for Rock Hard Abs or Young Living Oils). It's just about free books for those who appreciate my work, because I appreciate YOU. Simple as that.

Connect with Me

I welcome your questions, comments, and feedback of any kind. Please feel free to email me at joeylott@gmail.com. I am now receiving so many emails that I cannot always reply to every email. I do read them all, and I do my best to reply to as many as possible. For the benefit of others, I may choose to publish my response to your email on my blog or in book format. I will maintain your privacy and anonymity if I choose to publish my response.

One Small Favor

My sincere goal in writing is to share something that may be of value to you. And I endeavor to do so while keeping the costs low for readers. The success of my books and my ability to reach other readers who may benefit from my books depends in large part on having lots of thoughtful, honest reviews written about my work. You would do me a great favor if you would please take a moment to generously write a review of this book at Amazon.com. This will only take a few minutes of your time, and you will be helping me a great deal. I sure would appreciate it.

About the Author

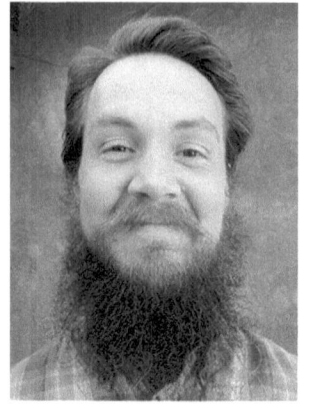

"The secret to happiness is to let go of everything - see through every assumption."

Beginning at a young age Joey Lott experienced intensifying anxiety. For several decades he lived with restrictive eating disorders, obsessions, compulsions, and an inescapable fear. By the time he was 30 years old he was physically sick, emotionally volatile, and mentally obsessed with keeping any and all unwanted thoughts and experiences at bay.

At this time Lott was living on a futon mattress in a tiny cabin in the woods. He was so sick that he could barely move. He was deeply depressed and hopeless. All this despite doing all the "right" things such as years of meditation, yoga, various "perfect" diets, clean air, and pure water.

Just when things were at their most dire, a crack appeared in the conceptual world that had formerly been mistaken for reality. By peering into this crack and underneath all the assumptions that had been unquestioned up to that moment, Lott began a great undoing. The revelation of this undoing is that reality is utterly simple, ever-present, seamless, and indivisible.

Lott's books provide a glimpse into the seamless, simple, and joyous nature of reality, offering a glimpse through the crack in conceptual worlds. Whether writing about the ultimate non-dual nature of reality, eating disorders, stress, disease, or any other subject, he offers the invitation to look at things differently, leaving behind the old, out-grown, painful limitations we have used to bind ourselves in suffering. And then, he welcomes you home to the effortless simplicity of yourself as you are.

Not sure where to begin? Pick up a copy of Lott's most popular book, You're Trying Too Hard, which strips away all the concepts that keep us searching for a greater, more spiritual, more peaceful life or self.

www.ingramcontent.com/pod-product-compliance
Lightning Source LLC
Chambersburg PA
CBHW050514290526
45786CB00007B/2557